Help Me Understand

What Happens When Someone in My Family Has Down Syndrome?

Jill and Sam Keppeler

PowerKiDS press™

New York

Published in 2020 by The Rosen Publishing Group, Inc.
29 East 21st Street, New York, NY 10010

First Edition

Editor: Rachel Gintner
Book Design: Rachel Rising

Photo Credits: Cover Maskot/Maskot/Getty Images; p. 4 Denis Kuvaev/Shutterstock.com; p. 5 Rawpixel.com/Shutterstock.com; p. 6 EstherQueen999/Shutterstock.com; pp. 7, 8 Monkey Business Images/Shutterstock.com; p. 10 Vol. Kozin/Shutterstock.com; p. 11 Monica Garza 73/Shutterstock.com; p. 12 Doro Guzenda/Shutterstock.com; p. 13 Eleonora_os/Shutterstock.com; p. 15 Syda Productions/Shutterstock.com; p. 17 AnnGaysorn/Shutterstock.com; p. 18 Denis Kuvaev/Shutterstock.com; p. 19 Ariel Skelley/DigitalVision/Getty Images; p. 21 digitalskillet/Shutterstock.com; p. 22 Gino Santa Maria/Shutterstock.com.

Cataloging-in-Publication Data

Names: Keppeler, Jill. | Keppeler, Sam.
Title: What happens when someone in my family has down syndrome? / Jill and Sam Keppeler.
Description: New York : PowerKids Press, 2020. | Series: Help me understand | Includes glossary and index.
Identifiers: ISBN 9781725309623 (pbk.) | ISBN 9781725309647 (library bound) | ISBN 9781725309630 (6 pack)
Subjects: LCSH: Down syndrome–Juvenile literature. | Down syndrome–Patients–Family relationships–Juvenile literature. | People with mental disabilities–Juvenile literature.
Classification: LCC RC571.K47 2020 | DDC 616.85'8842–dc23

Manufactured in the United States of America

CPSIA Compliance Information: Batch #CWPK20. For Further Information contact Rosen Publishing, New York, New York at 1-800-237-9932.

Contents

Everyone's Different

Everyone in this world is different. People have different hair colors, different skin colors, different smiles, and different shapes. Some people are tall. Some people are short. People also have different abilities and learn at different speeds.

Sometimes, people are born with a condition called Down syndrome. It's not a sickness, and it's not something you catch. Still, if you know and love someone with Down syndrome, you might wonder why they're a little different. Remember, though, they're mostly just like you!

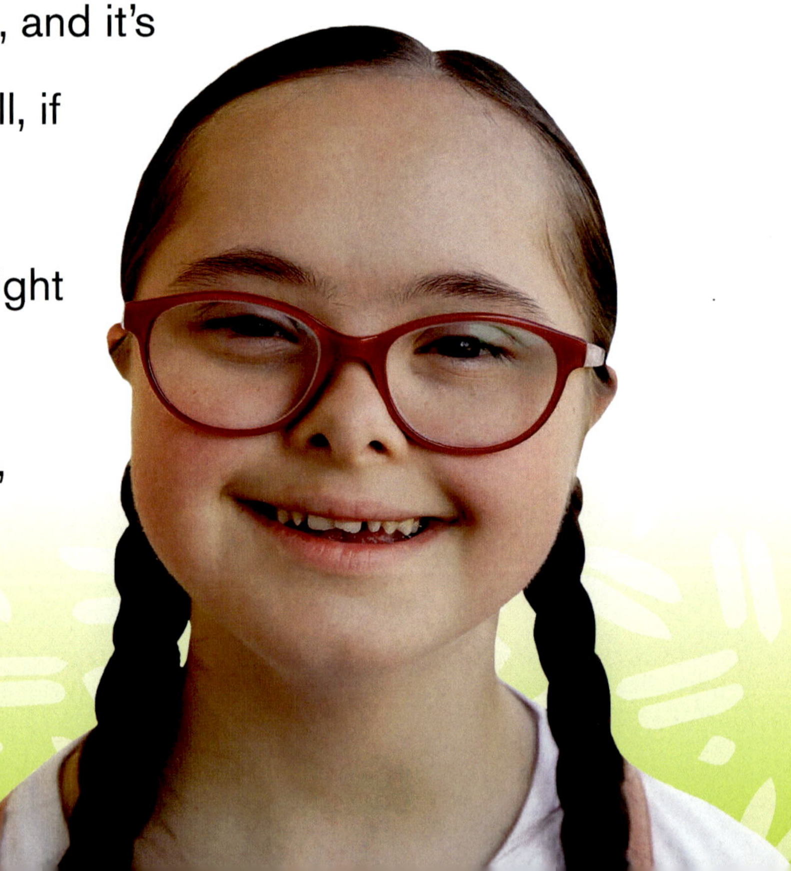

You might have a brother or sister with Down syndrome. They can still be your best friend!

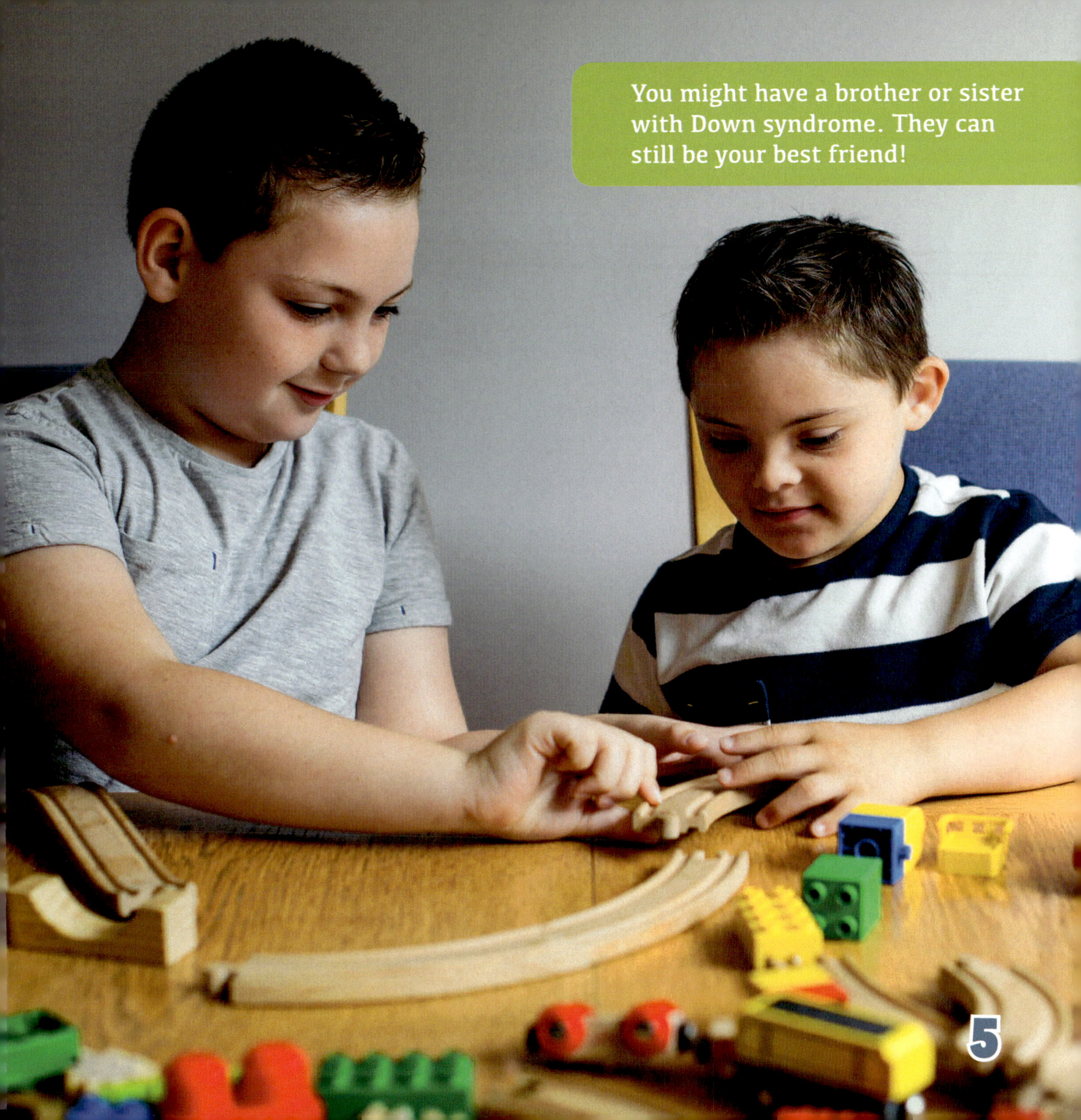

A Little Something Extra

People with Down syndrome are born with it. The condition has to do with chromosomes, which are parts inside every cell in your body. Chromosomes hold **genes**. Most people have 23 pairs of chromosomes, which means they have a total of 46.

However, people with Down syndrome have an extra chromosome, or an extra part of a chromosome, with the 21st set. Because of this, they're a little different. Their bodies form in a slightly different way.

chromosomes →

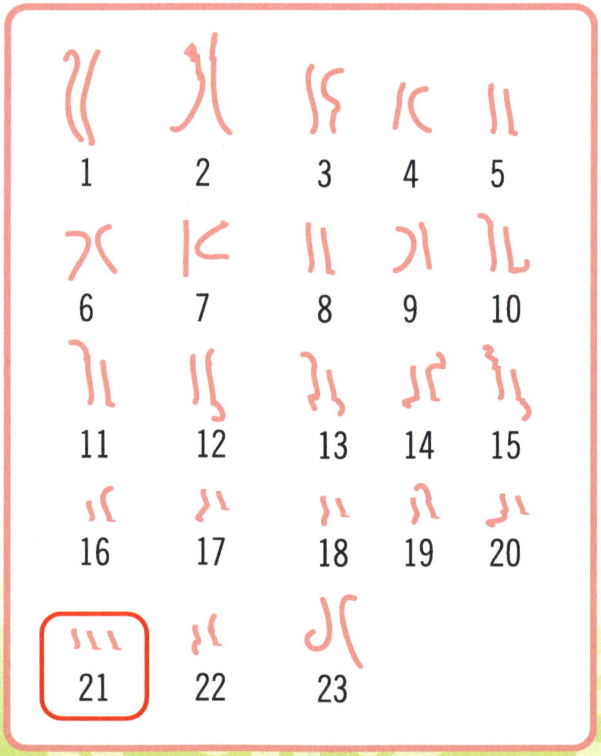

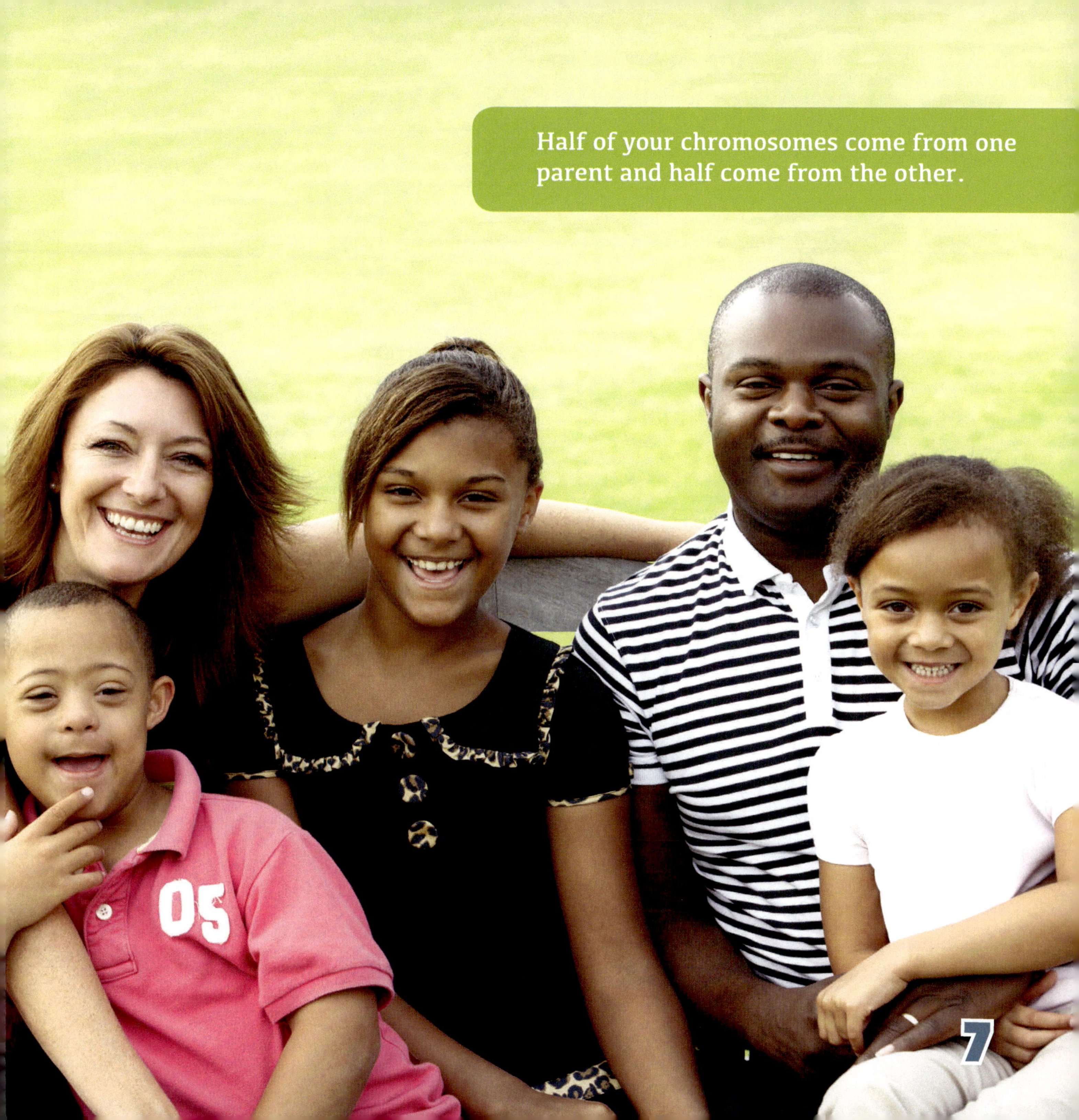

Half of your chromosomes come from one parent and half come from the other.

Health Problems

Because people with Down syndrome form differently before they're born, sometimes they have certain health issues. About half of all babies with Down syndrome are born with a heart problem. This means their heart doesn't work like it should. They might need **surgery** to fix it. This could be scary if it's your brother or sister.

Kids with Down syndrome may get sick more often. They might have problems hearing or seeing. They might need hearing aids or glasses—just like lots of other people.

People with Down syndrome often look a certain way. However, not all people with the condition will have the same **traits**.

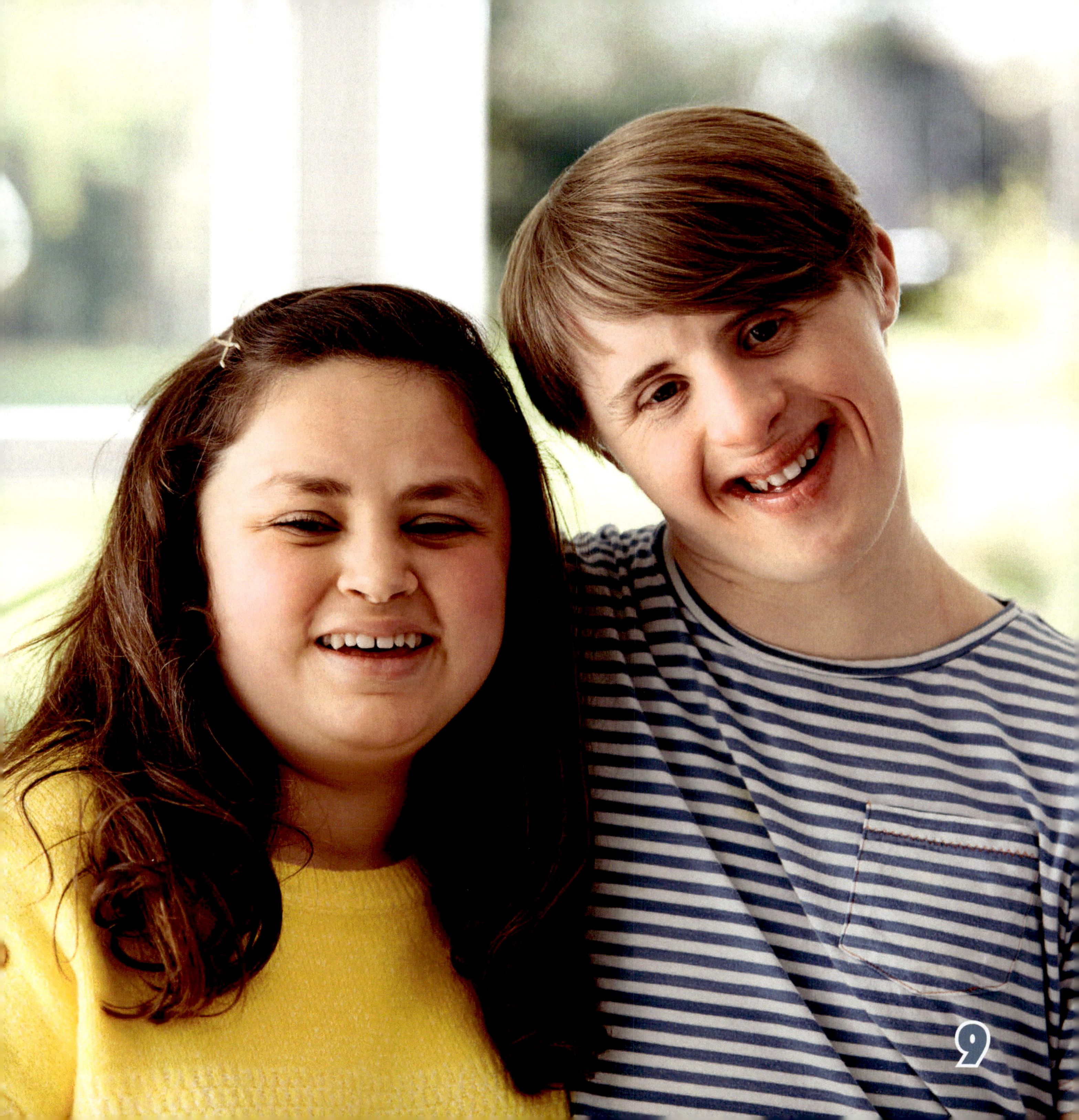

Their Own Path

If your family member with Down syndrome is a younger brother, sister, or cousin, you might be excited for them to get older. Maybe you can't wait to talk to them about things you like or to run and play with them.

However, children with Down syndrome often do things on a different timeline than children without it. They might talk later, walk later, or understand different things later. You might be **disappointed** because they can't play with you yet, but give them time and be **patient**.

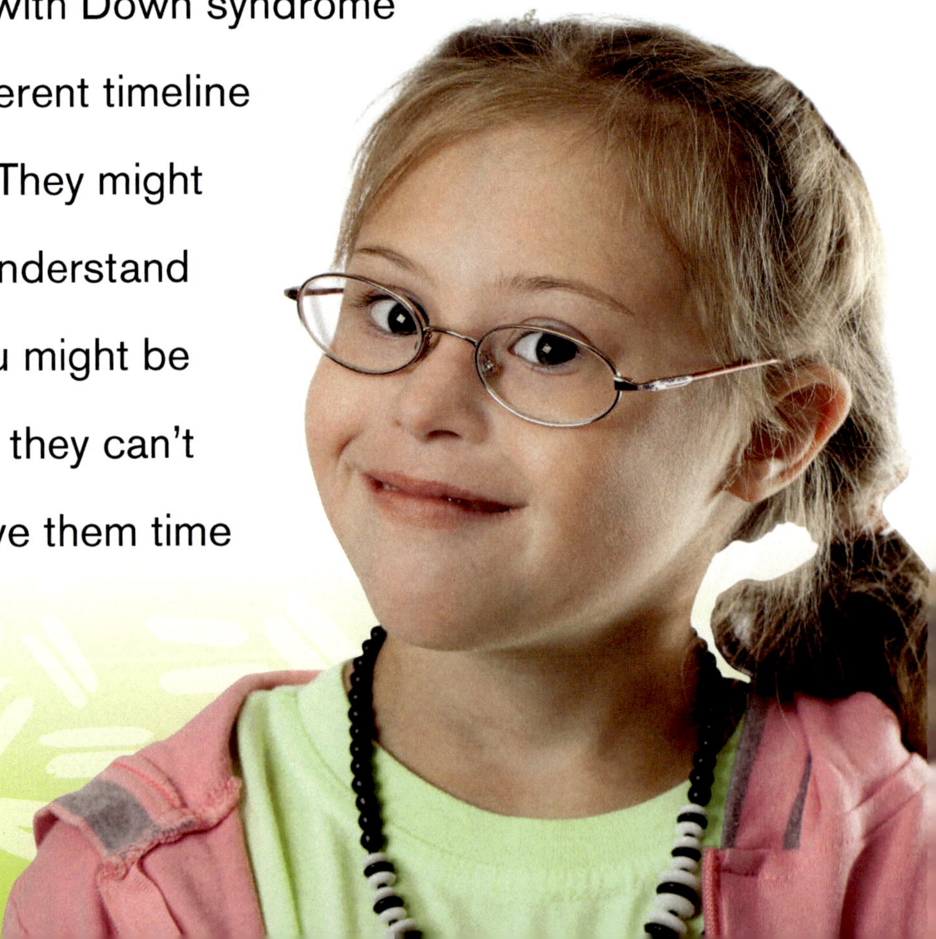

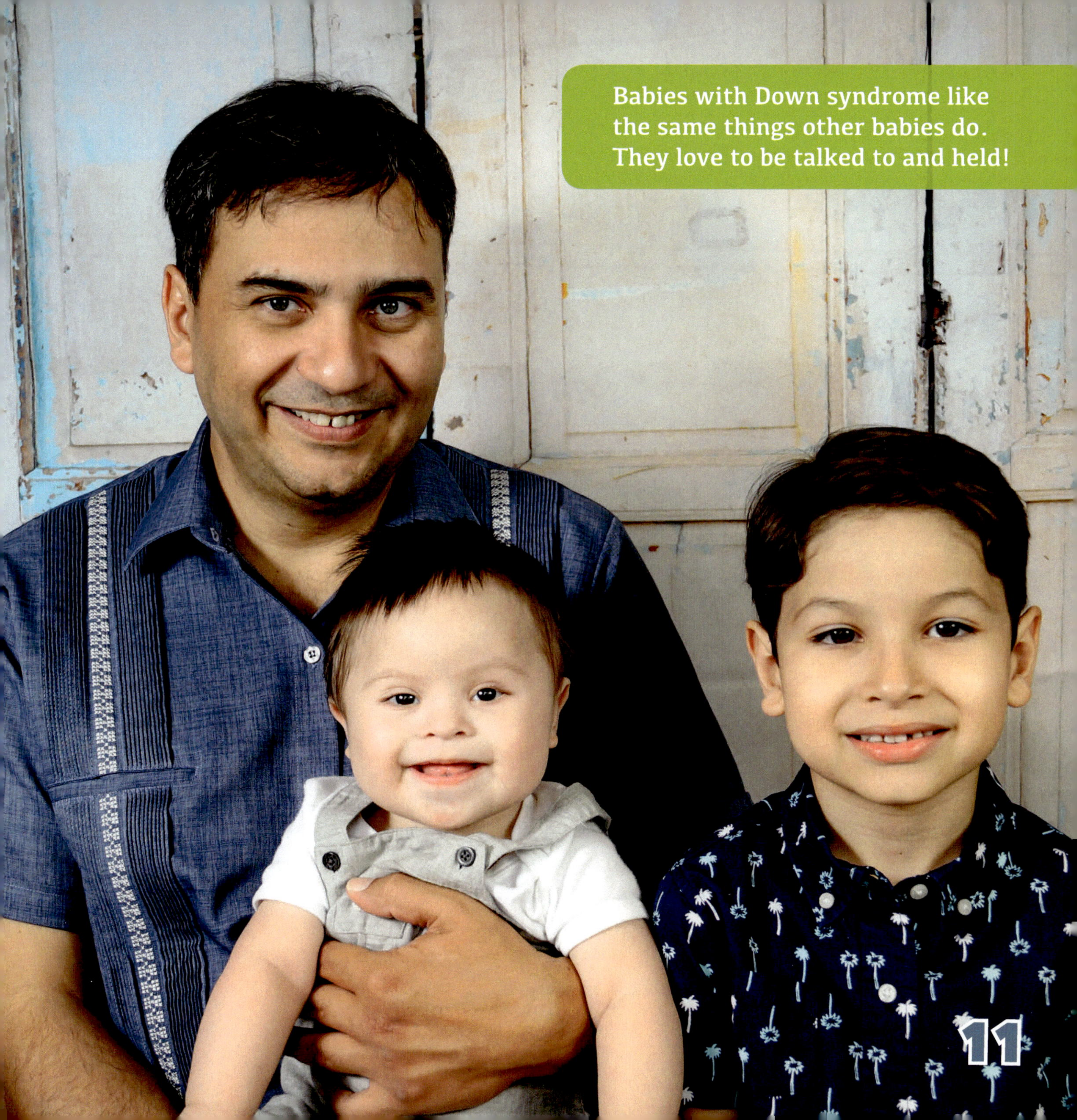

Babies with Down syndrome like the same things other babies do. They love to be talked to and held!

It's important to remember that your family member with Down syndrome will probably learn to do all or most of the things you can do. They might learn in a different way, and it might just take more time. You can show them all you can do!

Kids with Down syndrome go to school just like you. Maybe you know someone in your class with the condition. They might need a little extra help, but they still learn and play and take part.

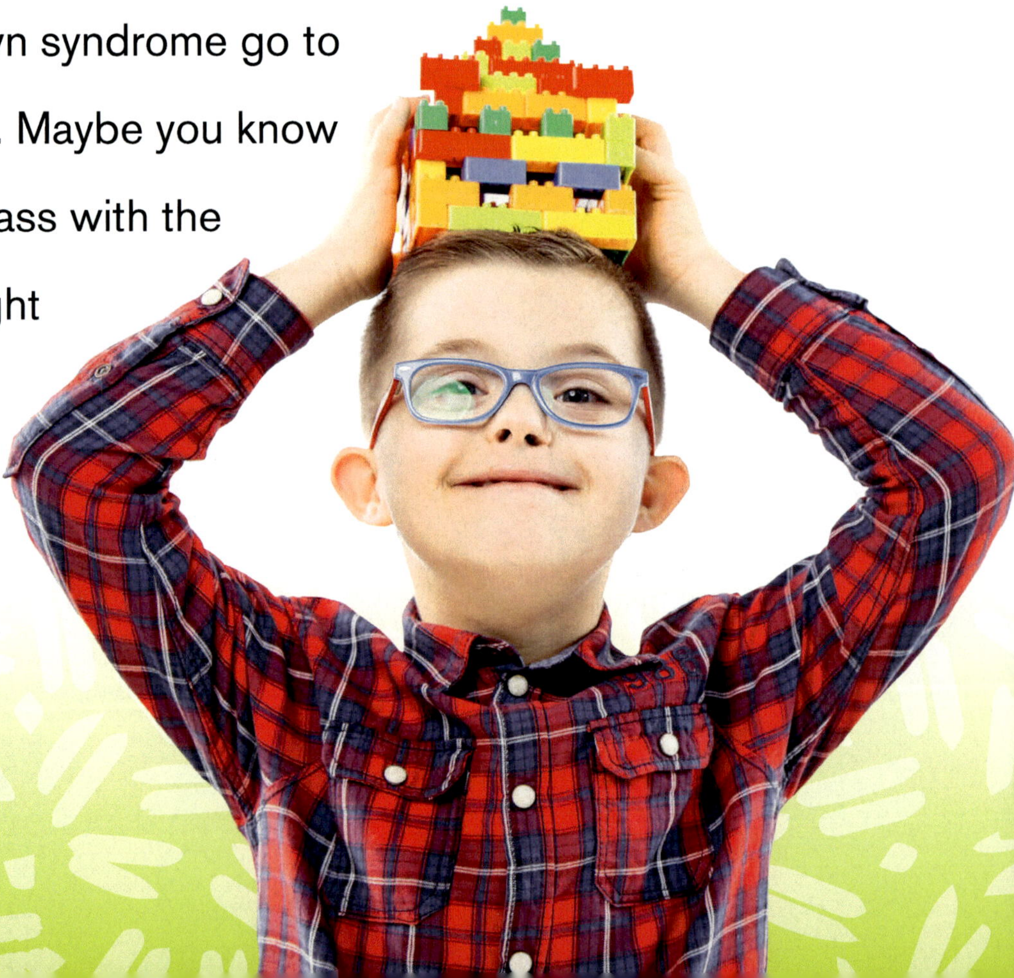

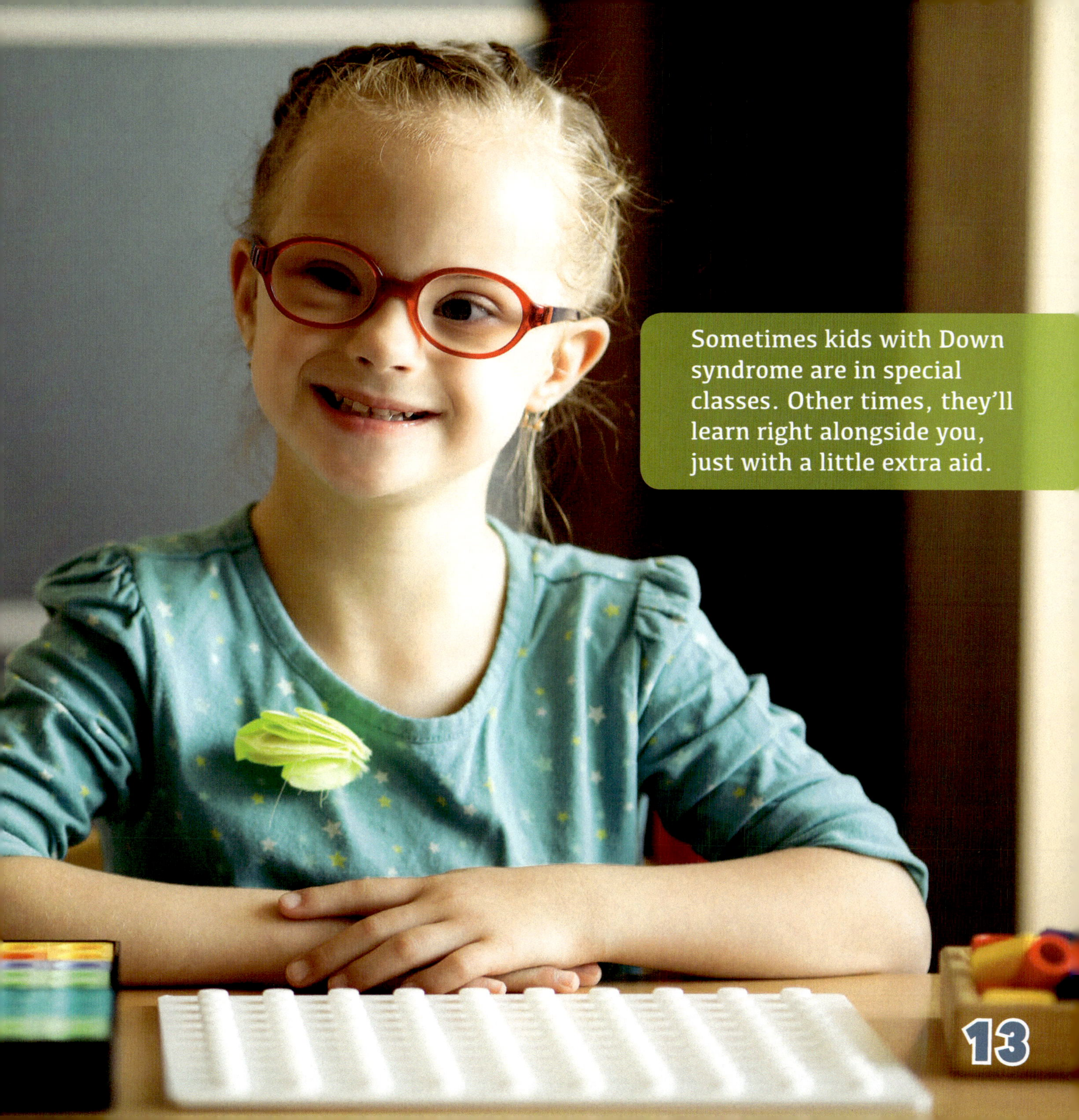

Sometimes kids with Down syndrome are in special classes. Other times, they'll learn right alongside you, just with a little extra aid.

Answering Questions

Because your family member with Down syndrome is different, your friends and classmates might ask questions about them. They might stare. They might even call them names! This may make you mad, sad, or even **embarrassed**. What do you do?

Be patient with your friends. They probably don't understand! Maybe they haven't been taught about Down syndrome. Explain why your family member is different. Remind your friends that they're more alike than they know and that people with Down syndrome have feelings, too.

Sometimes people can be mean. People who are your friends, though, will understand.

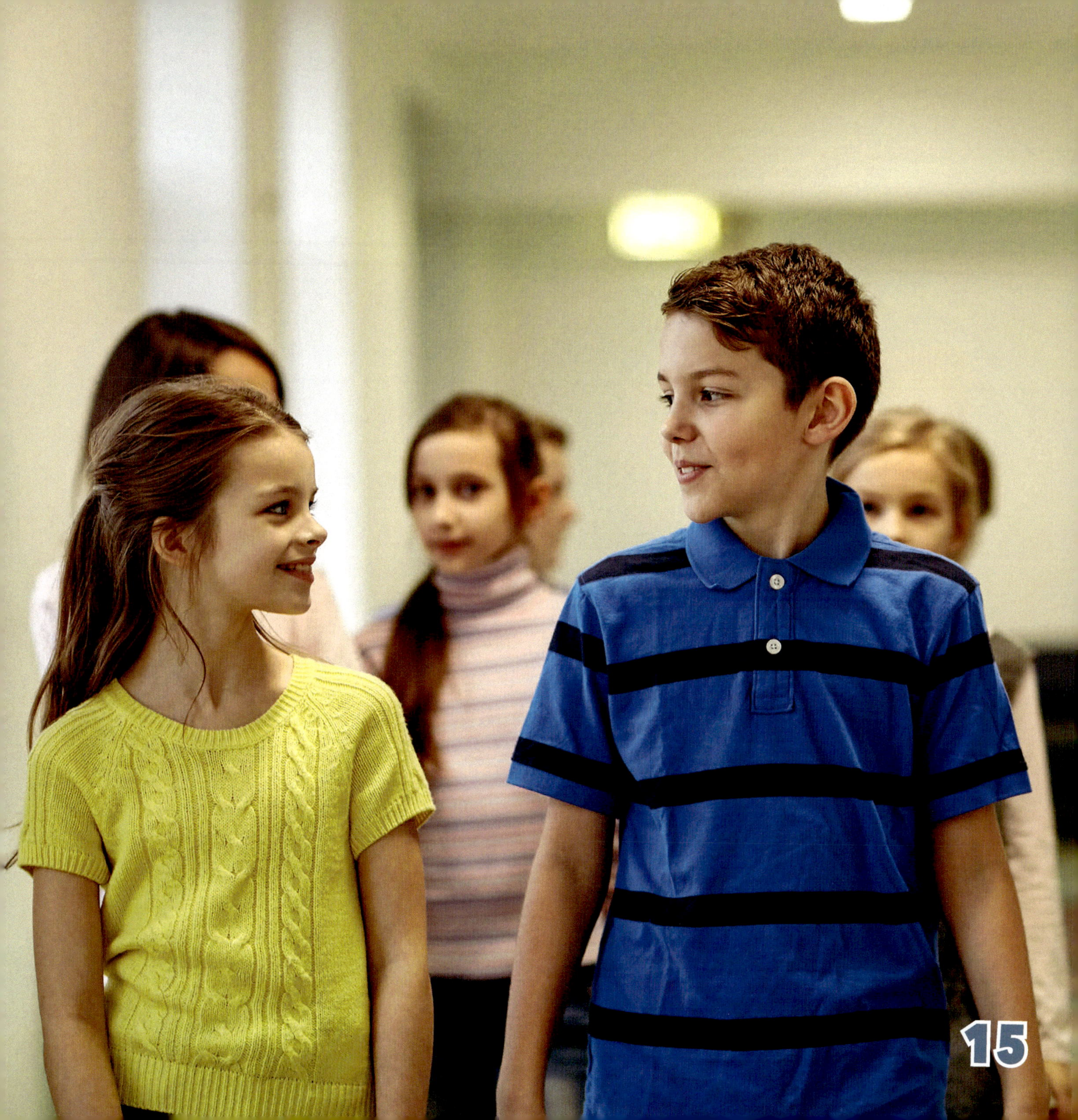

Sometimes, when you're out with your family, strangers might stare at your family member with Down syndrome. It could happen at a store, the library, or the park. Perhaps your brother or sister acts differently at times or has trouble with some situations. Maybe they don't always understand about being quiet or not saying certain things.

This might make you really upset! However, you can't teach everyone in the world, especially strangers. Try to **ignore** people when you can't talk to them about the problem.

There are a lot of **stereotypes** about people with Down syndrome. But they're just like everyone else—sometimes happy, sometimes sad, sometimes angry, sometimes silly!

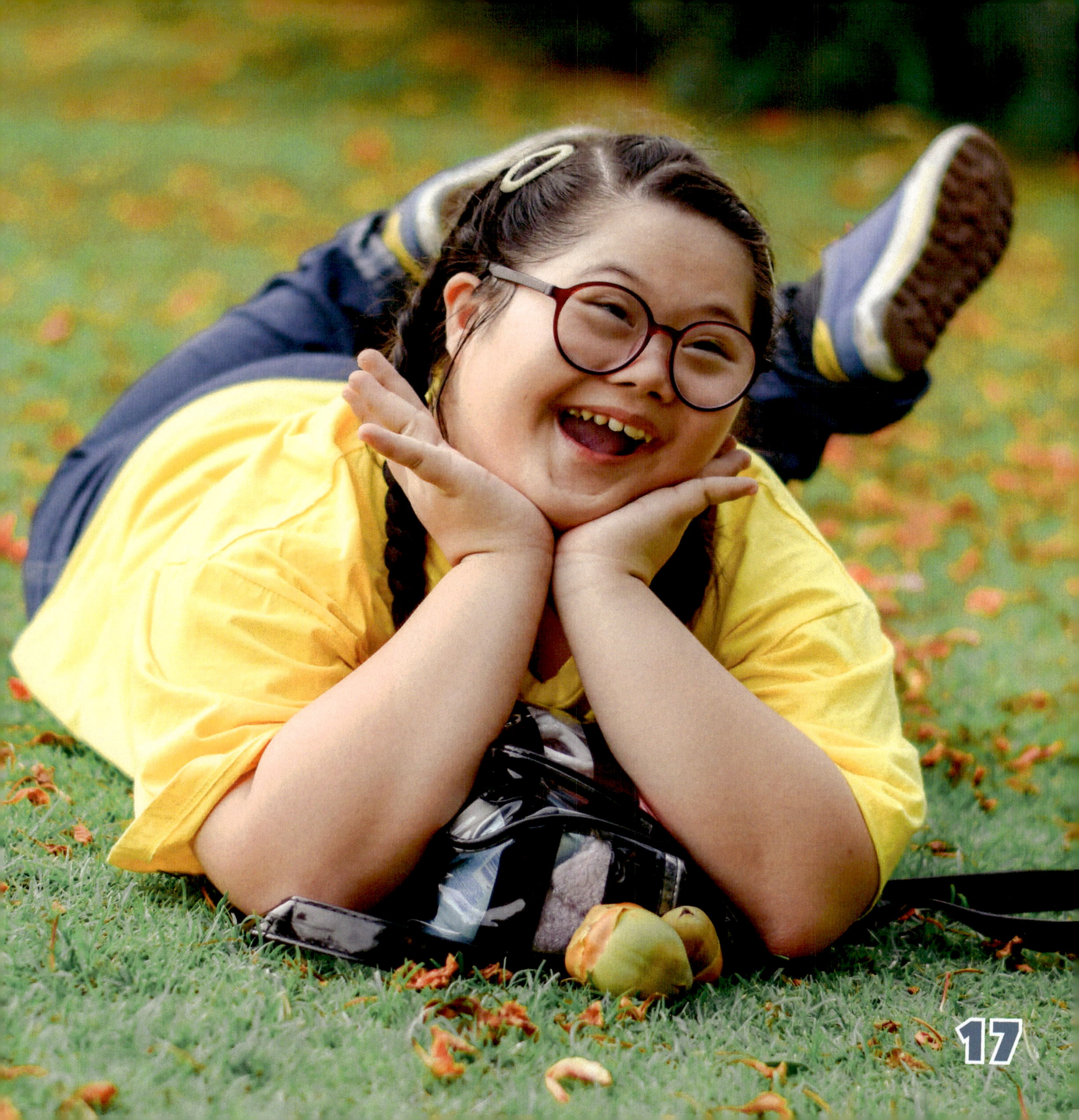

Being Patient

If you have a brother or sister with Down syndrome, you might have to be very patient with them. They might not understand things you think they should understand. They might not learn as fast as you would like. Sometimes, you might not be able to understand them.

Remember that they have feelings too, and they might be trying to understand and learn. Try to help them figure out things instead of getting upset that they're learning slowly.

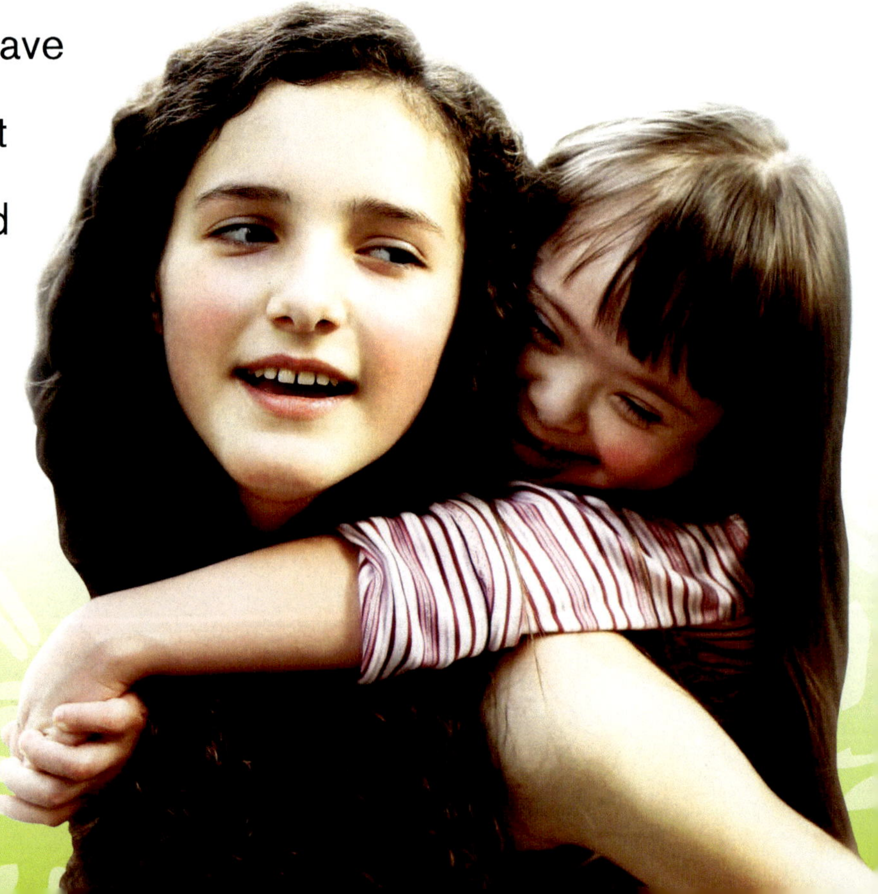

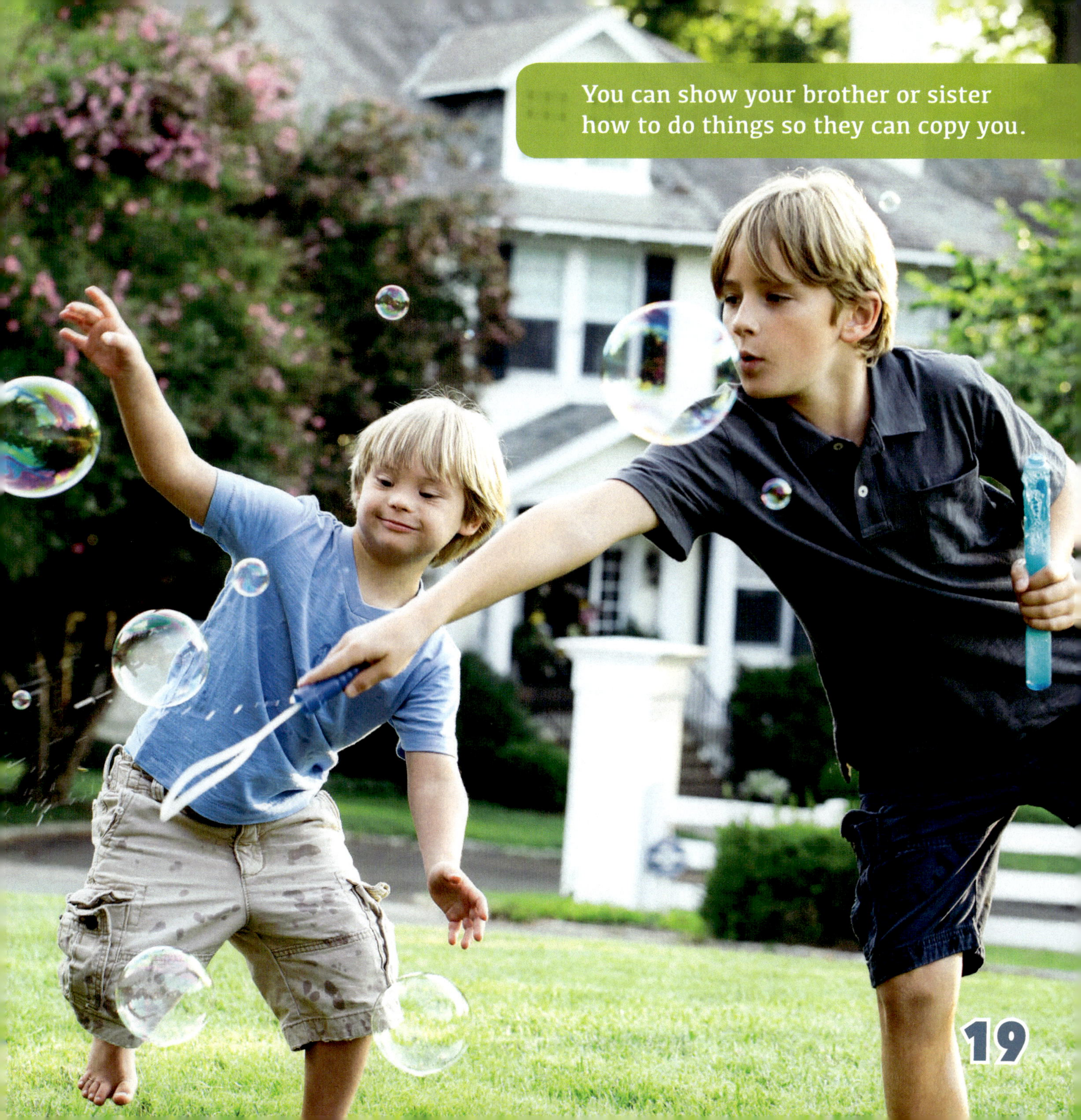

You can show your brother or sister how to do things so they can copy you.

I'm Frustrated!

No one can be patient all the time. Sometimes, you just might have had enough! Maybe your brother, sister, or cousin with Down syndrome broke something you own or made a big mess. It can be very **frustrating**, especially if they don't understand enough to fully clean up after themselves. Maybe you even have to help do it.

Take a deep breath. These feelings are **normal**! If you're really upset and frustrated, try to talk to your parents or another trusted adult about how you feel.

Maybe you need a break or some time alone with one of your parents. It's OK to tell them this.

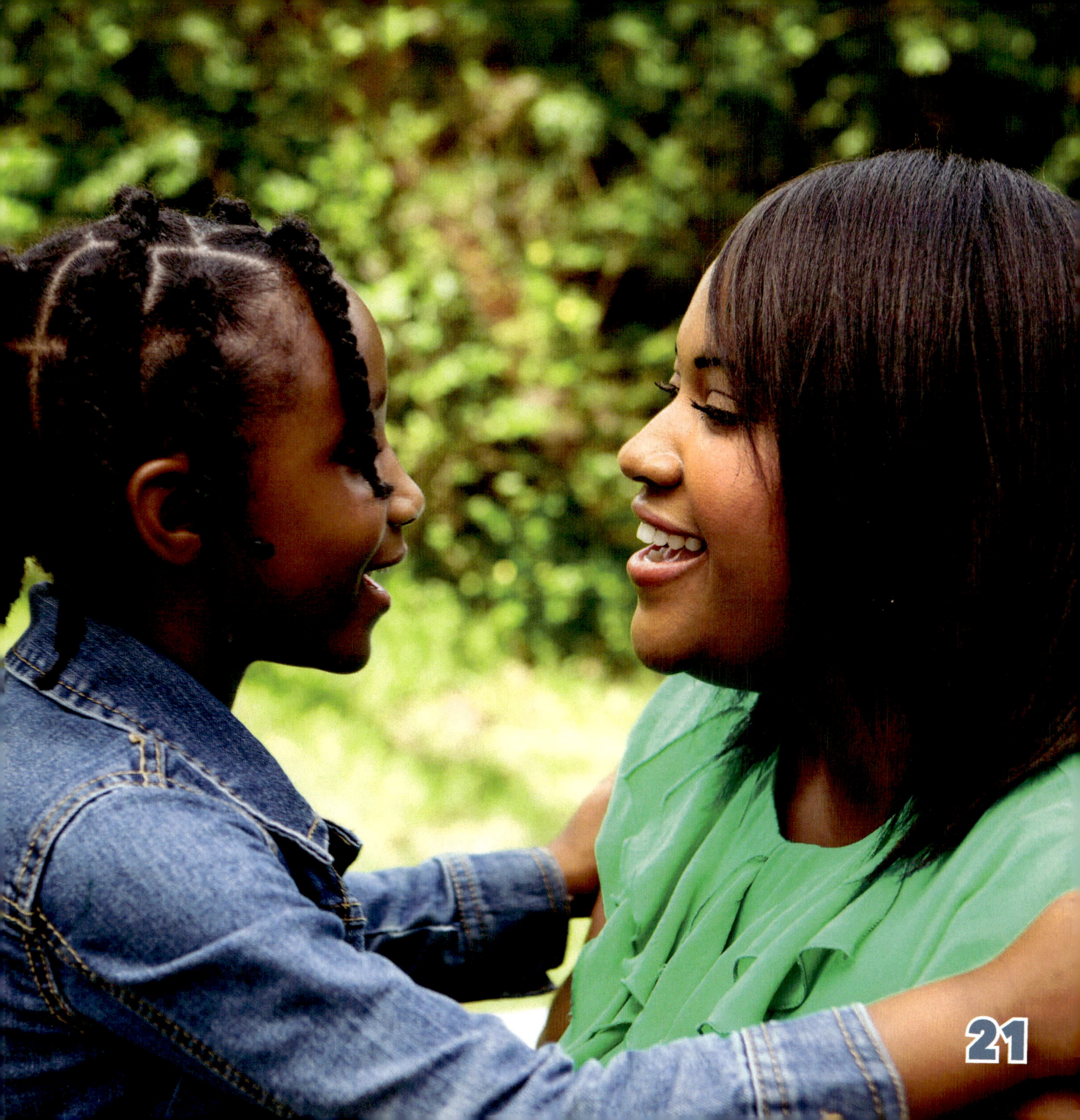

Helping Hands

People with Down syndrome often get some extra help. They might get **therapy** to help them learn how to speak and do other things. It's OK for you to need some help, too. Having a person with differences in the family can be a lot of work for everyone.

If you're having trouble or really want some more time and attention from your parents, just let them know. They'll want to give you what you need, too. Being a family is all about teamwork!

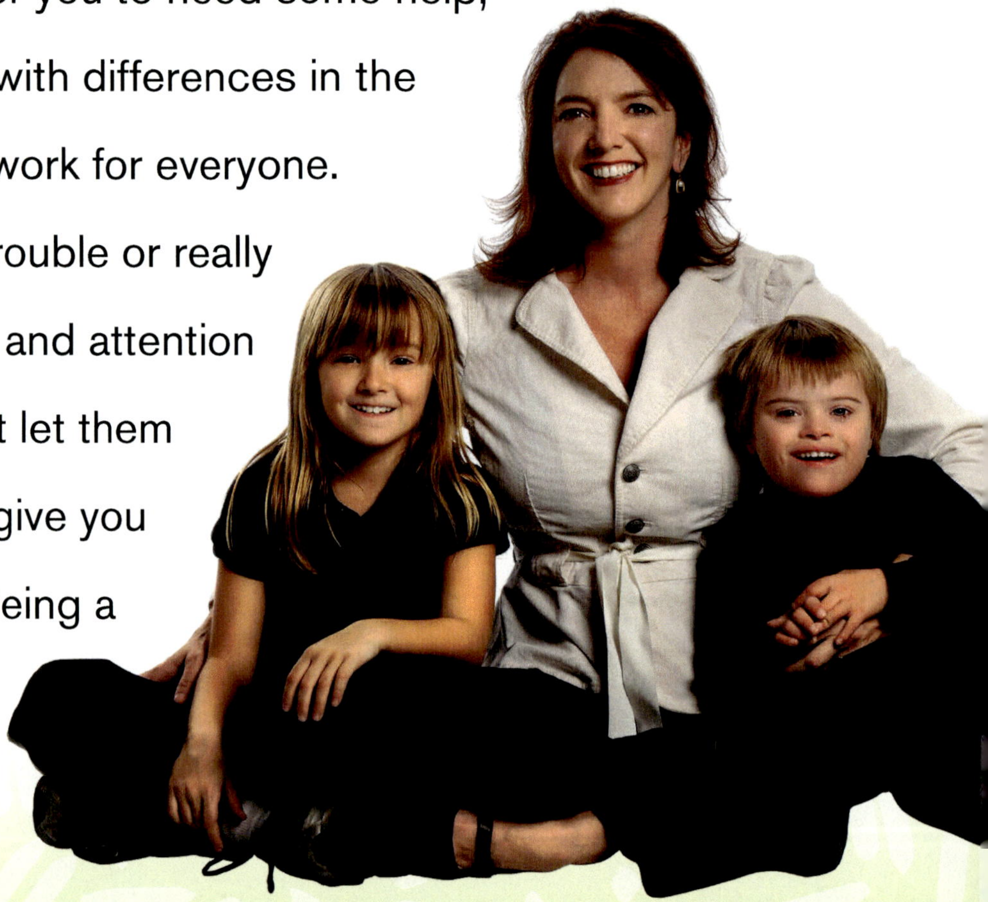

Glossary

disappointed: Feeling sad or unhappy because something isn't like you expected or wanted.

embarrassed: Feeling shame.

frustrating: Causing feelings of anger or being let down.

gene: A tiny part of a cell that's passed along from parent to child and decides certain features in the child, such as eye color.

ignore: To pay no attention to someone.

normal: Usual or ordinary.

patient: Able to remain calm when waiting a long time or dealing with problems.

stereotype: An unfair and often untrue belief that many people have about all people or things of a kind.

surgery: A medical treatment used for injuries and illnesses that involves operations.

therapy: A way of dealing with problems that makes people's bodies and/or minds feel better.

trait: A quality that makes one person or thing different from another.

Index

Websites

Due to the changing nature of Internet links, PowerKids Press has developed an online list of websites related to the subject of this book. This site is updated regularly. Please use this link toaccess the list: www.powerkidslinks.com/HMU/downsyndrome